WHAT NOW?

A SICK PERSON'S GUIDE
TO SURVIVING
THE UNITED STATES
OF AMERICA

by KEN BAUMANN

Copyright © 2021
Ken Baumann
kenbaumann.com

self-published via Amazon

ISBN: 9781737577607

Legal disclaimer: I'm not a medical professional. This book contains content provided for informational purposes only and is not intended as medical advice or as a substitute for the medical advice of a physician.

sickintheusa@protonmail.com

If you're sick, this book is for you.

If you're taking care of a sick person, this book is for you. If you're scared and confused and angry, this book is for you. If you want to know what it's like to struggle to stay alive in the United States of America, this book is for you.

I donate 10% of this book's proceeds to ripmedicaldebt.org, a charity "dedicated to removing the burden of medical debt for individuals and families and veterans across America."

TABLE OF CONTENTS

Intro ... 5
Map ... 9
Updates ... 10
Hospitals ... 11
— Tips & Tricks ... 11
— Going Home & Resting Up ... 17
— Bills & Prices ... 19
Meds ... 23
— Risks & Research ... 23
— Pharmacies & Insurance ... 26
Insurance ... 29
— Understanding the Terms ... 31
— Finding a Plan ... 34
— Using Your Coverage ... 36
— Fighting the Bullshit ... 38
— Covering Your Ass ... 41
Life ... 44
— Limits ... 45
— Fear ... 46
— Hope ... 47
Rules of Thumb ... 49
Resources ... 52

INTRO

I was twenty-two years old and about to get married when I needed to relearn how to walk.

A month earlier I had a steady job as an actor on a popular TV show. I was engaged to my favorite person. I had money, a house, a good dog, and a big appetite.

During meals I started feeling pain in my gut. One night the pain was so bad I quietly cried through a comedy show. Later that week I started limping. None of this made sense.

I went to a doctor I found on Yelp. He took an X-ray, recommended Chinese herbs, and sent me home.

I saw another doctor. When I told her I could barely eat and barely walk, she told me to go to the ER. Those doctors said I had a huge abscess on my psoas muscle that was probably about to burst. If that happened, they said, I might die.

In an hour my life completely changed. I struggled to breathe, eat, and defecate. I lived in a hospital bed. I felt the worst pain of my life, so bad I left my body. I needed help to do anything.

Everything.

I was diagnosed with Crohn's disease and prescribed steroids. I went home, took pills, and felt bad. I had to clean my bile and excrement out of a bag strapped to my stomach.

But the pills and waiting didn't work. I ran a 104° fever four nights in a row. A surgeon said he needed to operate. He hoped to do so with a laparoscope, a small device; he hoped that I'd recover quickly. He said a number that represented my chance of dying in the hospital (low, but real).

I sat in the car with my mom and fiance and told them what I wanted them to do if I died. The sun was bright. I remembered watching the trees sway in the wind.

The surgeons tried to use the small tools but found a big problem. They split my abdomen open, cut out 16 inches of my small intestine and colon, attached the new ends, then sewed me up.

I couldn't drink more than a few ounces of water for a day. I couldn't eat for three.

And then I needed to learn how to walk again.

My fiance held me as I walked up and down the bike path near our house every day at sunset. I could take a step every ten seconds. The first day I made it twenty feet. I kept practicing and she kept holding me.

I recovered.

Two months later we promised to love each other through sickness and through death. For us, this wasn't a hypothetical situation.

Then I started getting bills. Explanations of Benefits. Denied claims. Co-insurance charges. Prior Authorization requests and denials. The mail kept coming.

I'd grown up with sick parents, so I knew how bad our health care system can be. Now I know more about it. I say confidently that our health care system is cruel, crass, inefficient, fraudulent, arbitrary, and sickening. It makes us sicker. I watched this happen to my parents, and I experienced it happening to me. I watched the stress of it cause my dad to throw things through windows and my mom to scream in frustration and rage.

So I knew why the mail kept coming.

What I didn't know then—and what I had to learn the hard way—was what all the papers meant and how to deal with them. I didn't know how to survive in America as a sick person.

Ten years later, and with another disabling diagnosis on my resume (Major Depressive Disorder), I've learned a lot about how to navigate the terrible maze of American health care and health insurance. I've learned tricks, adopted rules of thumb, and followed principles that have literally kept me alive.

This book is for sick people, for their caretakers, and for those wise enough to know they'll one day be sick and need help.

I want to share all I know with you so that you don't suffer like I did. I want you to learn faster, adapt quicker, and get what you need more effectively than I did. I want this book to help you.

Because without help, being sick in the United States of America is a terminal condition.

MAP

I wrote this book to be read in an hour or two, but also to be referenced whenever you need it.

This book has four parts.

The first part, **HOSPITALS**, is about navigating those institutions. It'll explain how to protect yourself in them, how to find resources, and how to not get hustled.

The second part, **MEDS**, is about getting medicine in this country. It'll help you understand recommendations and risks, get the right meds at the right time, and define a bunch of jargon.

The third part, **INSURANCE**, will help you not give up when dealing with one of the USA's cruelest systems: health insurance companies and how they treat people. It'll explain how these companies operate and teach you methods you can use to beat them at their own game.

The fourth part, **LIFE**, is short. It summarizes what I've learned while trying to survive in the USA as a sick person. It's also about what we could do to make society kinder to the sick and the poor. I hope the last part leaves you hopeful.

UPDATES

I update this book as I learn more. Those changes are listed here: kenbaumann.com/blog/what-now-changelog

If you've bought a paperback copy and want an updated ebook edition, please email me a proof of purchase.

If you're chronically ill and want to share advice, please tell me. If you work for a health insurance company and want to share info, please tell me. If you're a medical professional and want to guide patients, please tell me.

I can credit you or leave you anonymous.

Up to you.

sickintheusa@protonmail.com

HOSPITALS

If you entered the American health care system under big red letters that say *EMERGENCY*, the most important thing you can do is try to heal.

This means different things for different people. If you're sick right now, so sick that reading and thinking is difficult, give this book to someone you trust then ask them to help you.

If you're in the hospital alone, I know how scary this can be. Try to get a close friend or family member to stay with you and help you make decisions and deal with doctors, nurses, and other hospital staff. Email this book or hand it to them.

Your only responsibility right now is to stay alive and trust yourself.

TIPS & TRICKS

If you're recovering and can read this comfortably, great. I'm happy you're healing.

Hospitals can feel stuck in time, but there are moments in hospitals that will shape your path as a sick person. Being prepared for these moments is vital.

First: ask someone you trust to stay with you. Ideally this is a close friend or family member, but someone is better than no one.

RULE OF THUMB #1: Ask someone you trust to help. Having someone who can advocate for you, listen, and guide your decisions will make your life as a sick person much easier.

Once you have someone to help, ask them to do the following tasks:
1. Write everything down.
2. Ask questions if something doesn't make sense.
3. Get attention when you need it.
4. Google stuff.
5. Be nice until you need to be terrifying.

Some people are uncomfortable in hospitals, but your helper might have fun. Why? Because navigating a hospital's challenges intelligently and efficiently can feel like beating a hard video game. It's thrilling to help someone in a complex environment.

If you can't get someone you know to help, ask your nurses to bring you a patient advocate. If the hospital doesn't have one, ask your boss or Human Resources person at work if their benefits plan includes patient advocates. Or you can hire a private patient advocate (like those provided by patientadvocate.org).

Finally, if those options don't work for you, many nurses will happily help you. You can ask them to write things down for you, ask questions, and Google stuff. They won't be able to help all the time, but a little help can go a long way.

Here are details about each of your helper's tasks:

1. Write everything down.

Every time a medical professional says something that's not small talk, write it down. Names of medications, possible diagnoses, confirmed diagnoses, procedures, tests, addresses, names of doctors: everything.

Doctors tend to be busy and distracted, so ask doctors to repeat, explain, and spell any words you don't know. If the doctor is talking too fast, ask them to slow down. If they say something that contradicts what another medical professional said, tell them that.

You want to make sure your medical professionals aren't working against each other or misunderstanding the sick person's situation.

Be nice, calm, and logical. Don't tolerate dismissive attitudes.

Not dying as a sick person is hard and serious work, so doctors should be as serious and patient as possible. You might need to remind doctors that this is their responsibility.

RULE OF THUMB #2: Write everything down. Whenever you talk with someone who has power over your health and finances, write down their name, contact info, the date, and what they say. You can use this info later to protect yourself.

2. Ask questions if something doesn't make sense.

If something doesn't make sense, ask questions until it does. If the person you're talking to can't answer your questions, get them to connect you to someone who does.

Often in hospitals nurses know more about patients than doctors since nurses spend more time with them. Use your nurses' knowledge while talking with doctors.

If you don't know who to ask for info, call a nurse or walk to the nearest nurse's station. State your question clearly and calmly. It might help to write it down beforehand. Follow up until you're given a clear answer.

3. Get attention when you need it.

Sick people in hospital beds can press a little button (a green one, in my experience) that calls a nurse.

Sometimes these buttons send that call to Jupiter; sometimes nurses are busy with other patients in worse conditions.

This doesn't mean you should be ignored.

If you're in pain and want to feel better, ask a nurse to help.

If you feel something new or unusual, ask a nurse to help.

If you need help doing something—like sitting up or going to the bathroom—ask a nurse to help.

If you need to contact someone but don't know how, ask a nurse to help.

Nurses are some of the best people on the planet. Some are assholes, exhausted, or bad at their jobs because humans are fallible. But in my experience most nurses are nurses because they enjoy helping people.

So don't feel afraid, nervous, or ashamed to get attention. If you need it and aren't getting it in a reasonable timeframe, cause a fuss. You can always apologize later. (More on that soon.)

4. Google stuff.

The medical field, like all scientific fields, is full of technical jargon and people who magically believe that everyone else knows the same terms.

Living in a hospital is like learning a new language. And fast.

If a doctor says you might have Disease X, Google it. Read about it from reputable sources (often big hospitals' websites, though WebMD and Wikipedia are often fine). Write down what's relevant to the sick person's experience and what isn't. You can bring up those notes when you talk with your doctor and nurse.

Using the internet to research your situation is a basic survival skill. As a sick person or sick person's helper, you need to be comfortable researching stuff on the internet.

Trust your judgement, find reputable sources, and learn when you can. The more you can learn about your condition while you're in the hospital, the better.

5. Be nice until you need to be terrifying

Most people mean well. Most medical professionals will try to help you. If you show them appreciation and kindness, they will often work harder to help you.

The old saying that you catch more flies with honey than vinegar, or that you get more with sugar than salt, is true. We're all mirrors and mimics.

But sometimes being nice doesn't work in a stressful, complicated, and confusing environment—like a hospital. Sometimes your kindness and patience will be ignored.

And sometimes you'll need to not be ignored—because you're in pain, you're scared, or because someone is telling you to do what you know you shouldn't (like take the wrong medication, or move when someone told you to rest, or get a test done that you already got done.)

When that happens, you need to become terrifying.

In the hospital, this means doing some or all of the following:

- Using imperative language ("Get me my medicine now.")
- Shouting.
- Showing your anger.
- Using bureaucratic threats (like filing a complaint to your state's medical board).
- Annoying people until they give up their other work and prioritize you.
- Demanding a second or third opinion from another medical professional.

When you're in this mode, don't budge until you get what you need.

RULE OF THUMB #3: Be nice, but use anger as a tool. Sadly, anger can more effectively get you attention from people with power. As a sick person, though, anger can make you sicker—so use it wisely.

GOING HOME & RESTING UP

Once you've healed enough to go home, you'll be "discharged." (This means you'll be made to leave.) Before you leave the hospital, it will help

you to have:
- Your final diagnoses
- Your prescribed medicines and doses
- What not to eat, drink, and do while healing
- What you should eat, drink, and do while healing
- What signs of healing to look for
- What signs of getting sicker to look for
- Followup appointments
- The name and number of who to call with questions
- The names and titles of other doctors you're being referred to
- The phone number and email address of the hospital's billing department
- Info about the hospital's charity care or financial assistance program
- A copy of your complete medical records (digital and paper)
- Ideally, a business card of a hospital executive or someone else "higher up"

RULE OF THUMB #4: Work with people with fancier-sounding job titles. They have more power and information so they can help you more efficiently. Keep their contact info handy.

Once you're home, your primary goal is to rest and heal.

Because the American federal government treats working people poorly, many working class people don't have the right to take paid time off. This means your boss might expect you to return to work right away.

I can't ethically tell you what to do in that situation. What I do know, though, is that you can't rush healing and can't force yourself to be better. There's no substitute for restful time in a safe and comfortable environment. This might mean that it'll be better for your health in the longterm to quit your job and collect unemployment benefits.

Being healthy is the foundation on which life's best moments are often built. Sometimes jobs prevent you from being healthy. Talk with your loved ones about your priorities.

BILLS & PRICES

A senior doctor at a huge hospital system told me a story about medical prices.

He said back in the 80's, Saudi oil barons would fly to his hospital for medical treatment. To pay for the hospital's services, they would break out scales and measure their payments in gold. Actual gold.

His hospital's bosses quickly learned that these oil barons would pay whatever prices they were charged.

The doctor then told me that medical prices in

that hospital system were set for everyone based on those pay-in-gold rates.

Whether this story is true or not, medical prices in the US are scarily high. And they're going up. But we must remember that these prices are set by human beings.

There's an open secret known by hospital billing departments and insurance companies everywhere: all medical bills are negotiable. You can pick a fight about whatever bill is thrown at you.

RULE OF THUMB #5: Bills are negotiable. They're made by people and people can be persuaded to change their minds. Don't panic.

Many hospitals are nonprofit, and "[under] the Affordable Care Act, nonprofit hospitals[...] are required to provide free or discounted care to patients of meager incomes — or risk losing their tax-exempt status[.]" [khn.org/news/patients-eligible-for-charity-care-instead-get-big-bills/] What this means is that many hospitals have forms online you can fill out to lower your bills—sometimes to $0. Ask people in the hospital's billing department to refer you to their financial assistance/charity care policy.

If you don't qualify for charity care because your income is too high, remember that no bill is inevitable. You can call the hospital's billing department and negotiate a better price and/or a monthly payment plan. Keep at it. Persuasion works.

Before doing this, though, the first thing to do when you get a big bill from a hospital or medical provider is ask for a line-item bill. Most bills are vague; some hide outrageous charges (like $100 for a bag of saltwater or $40 for two Tylenols). Line-item bills show you those charges. You can use that info in your conversations with the billing department.

Some bills show what your insurance company has paid towards them. If that number doesn't make sense, call your insurance company and ask for an explanation. (More on that in the **INSURANCE** section.)

Newly sick people often get bills from a ton of different providers. This can be confusing. Why does it happen? Because some medical providers (like anesthesiologists) are independent contractors, so they bill patients directly. Double-check that you're not getting double-billed for the same service.

RULE OF THUMB #6: Don't pay medical bills immediately. Bills say how long you have to pay them (it's usually 30, 60, or 90 days). First understand and negotiate those charges and prices.

This rule of thumb has an important followup:

RULE OF THUMB #7: Value your time. Waiting on hold for hours can be as harmful as a disease's symptoms, so figure out what your time is worth per hour. Use that number to choose which bills you fight.

MEDS

$47,684.

That's how much my insurance company paid for one dose of the drug I take for Crohn's disease.

$6,280.

That's what my insurance company billed me for that same dose.

As a sick person, you'll need medicine to survive. Sadly for folks who live in the United States, this need is a financial burden—and fulfilling this need can be a threat to our mental health.

On top of that, most people can't completely understand the risks of taking most drugs.

I'll walk you through the common obstacles between you and your medicine, as well as some helpful ways to consider which medications are right for you.

RISKS & RESEARCH

If you enter the US health care system through an ER, you probably won't get to choose which drugs you're prescribed. Doctors and nurses work fast and prefer some drugs over others (sometimes for unethical reasons), and you won't have time to talk through options in a medical emergency.

Once you've recovered enough to talk with your doctors and nurses, find out which drugs you've been given. (Or have your helper find out.) Write them down.

Once you've healed up some more, research online the drugs you're expected to keep taking. Find out how long your doctors expect you to take them, and research the risks of taking those meds longterm.

Here's some jargon to watch out for:

- **Indications**: this means that the FDA (Food and Drug Administration) believes a drug is effective in treating a given disease, so its manufacturer has legal permission to market the drug that way. (For example: Remicade is indicated to treat moderately to severely active Crohn's disease and rheumatoid arthritis.)
- **Side effects**: Note a drug's most dangerous/severe side effects as well as its most common. Find percentages of people who've suffered those side effects. These symptoms and numbers can help you pick medications.
- **Warnings & Precautions**: this usually refers to the worst possible side effects of taking a drug.
- **Drug interactions**: Many drugs interact with other drugs. Human bodies are complex; it's

usually safer to make fewer changes to complex systems. So it's usually safer to take as few drugs as possible.

- **Contraindications**: situations in which certain people shouldn't take a drug. For example, if you suffer from moderate to severe heart failure, you shouldn't take Remicade (because you're much more likely to experience life-threatening side effects). Double and triple check with your medical professionals that you don't fit a category of a drug's contraindications.

All the terms above show up in every drug's medication guide and all medicines have one. Try to read the guides of the drugs your medical professionals want to prescribe you. Talk with folks you trust about the risks and requirements. Ask your insurance for costs.

Lastly, consider how often you'll need to take the drug in question, because "it is estimated that adherence to chronic medications is about 50%." [uspharmacist.com/article/medication-adherence-the-elephant-in-the-room] (*Adherence* means a person taking the right amount of their prescribed medications on schedule.) Sadly, "[nonadherence] can account for up to 50% of treatment failures, around 125,000 deaths, and up to 25% of hospitalizations each year in the United States."

Set up a schedule or routine to take your meds. I have an alarm on my phone that rings twice a day to remind me to take Wellbutrin and calendar alerts twice a month to schedule my next Remicade infusion.

RULE OF THUMB #8: When in doubt, take your time.

If your condition allows you to, research drugs and their risks, ask questions, and make a careful and deliberate decision.

PHARMACIES & INSURANCE

Expensive drugs are harder to get. Ask your hospital's billing department what the hospital typically bills a common insurance company for a dose, or do some Googling to see what other patients pay. (Keep in mind that hospitals often charge more for drugs than pharmacies.)

Every health insurance plan has a formulary. This is a list of drugs they'll pay for, try their damndest not to pay for (usually calling them "non-preferred" and/or a "speciality medication"), and a list of drugs they won't touch with a ten foot pole (called "non-formulary" and/or a "speciality medication").

If you've got health insurance, call and email the company and/or its pharmacy benefits manager. Ask for a plain written statement of their policies on each drug you need. (Doctors usually make sure your insurance plan covers the drugs they prescribe you, but since "cover" can mean anything from "pay 100% of the cost" to "anything over $100 is your responsibility, buddy!", do your research.)

Expensive drugs are associated with my least favorite two-word phrase in the English language: Prior Authorization.

A Prior Authorization, or PA, is basically a big metal door and a mean-looking guard keeping you from entering a party you've been invited to. PA requests are one of the main tricks that health insurance companies use to not "lose" money on the sick people they claim to help. If your insurance company hates paying for a particular drug, they'll require your medical providers to send them a PA request. Your provider will need to send your insurance company documents that show that a) you need the drug, b) it's the best option for you, and c) it's helping you heal or preventing you from getting sicker.

Prior Authorizations usually last six months to a year. This means that some drugs in the United States of America come with the additional requirement of begging your insurance company to keep paying for your life. The PA process can be humiliating, frustrating, and fraudulent. Keep this in mind when choosing medications.

Finally, co-pay assistance programs might be available through your medications' manufacturers, as well as health insurance companies and pharmacies. These programs usually provide a fixed amount of money to you each year that you can use to pay co-pays and other out-of-pocket costs.

INSURANCE

Every time my health insurance company calls me I feel sick to my stomach.

Dealing with health insurance companies in the United States is miserable. Even with great coverage, even with plenty of money, it will sap your energy and make you feel worse.

Why? There are many reasons, but here are a few.

On the one hand, many health insurance companies are for-profit corporations. They make money off healthy people (by collecting more money in charges than they pay out for claims) and lose money off sick people (by paying out more money in claims than they collect in charges). For-profit companies are built to enrich their owners and sick people are more costly, thus sick people are liabilities to health insurance companies. These companies have a huge incentive to not pay for what you need.

On the other hand, health insurance companies like when they're charged high prices. Why? Because they can use those prices to justify increasing their charges to their customers.

Before the Affordable Care Act was signed into law, health insurance companies could spend however much or however little of the money they charged in premiums on their customers' medical care. A provision in the ACA makes them spend 80–85% of the money they make from customers' premiums on actual health care—not on executive salaries and TV commercials.

Insurance industry insiders have a name for the percentage of income they're legally obligated to spend on their customers: the "Medical Loss Ratio." This gross phrase reveals health insurance companies' attitude towards sick people.

Another reason why dealing with health insurance companies is exhausting is that health insurance companies offer tens, hundreds, or even thousands of health insurance plans—and each "covers" certain medical professionals, hospitals, and drugs and doesn't cover all others. (Sick people need to always know who is "in-network.") Other wealthy countries are smarter than us, offering health insurance through their governments or heavily regulating insurance companies so that they can't wreck people's lives to increase their profits.

Regardless of the history and reasons, this is our reality (until we convince our Congresspeople to improve Medicare and offer it to every person, regardless of age—or change our medical system in some other big way). If you're chronically ill, you're going to deal with health insurance companies until the day you die. This is scary, frustrating, and sad. I know. I'm sorry.

But there are a few things you can learn and a few tricks you can use to make dealing with them easier.

UNDERSTANDING THE TERMS

Insurance doesn't need to be complicated. Think about a life insurance policy: you pay the insurance company small amounts of money every month in the understanding that when you die, they'll pay your family a bigger amount. Pay in when times are good, get paid when times are bad. Simple.

But when you compare health insurance policies, you'll face all kinds of vague and boring words, phrases, and acronyms: coinsurance, copay, deductible, premium, coverage, provider, formulary, maximum out-of-pocket, HMO, PPO, out-of-network. It goes on and on. I'll define the most important terms in everyday language below.

Let me first summarize what American health insurance companies do:

If you pay them each month, visit only the facilities and professionals they approve, and use the drugs they want you to, then they will sometimes pay for those goods and services.

Most health insurance companies provide a bad service for a high price. And make billions of dollars in profit every year.

As a sick person, I've learned to enjoy not letting them screw me. Hopefully you can too.

- **Coinsurance**: charges your company won't pay for. Usually it's a percentage of the total charge. (Example: if your policy says you'll owe a 20% coinsurance on specialty prescription drugs, they'll expect you to pay 20% of the price they're charged.)
- **Copay**: what you need to pay medical providers when you use their services. (Example: if your policy says you have a $50 copay for seeing specialists, those offices will charge you $50 before seeing a doctor.)
- **Deductible**: what you have to spend each year before the insurance company pays for anything. (Example: if your policy has a $5,000 deductible, you'll be expected to pay $5,000 for health care before the insurance company begins to maybe pay for stuff.)
- **Premium**: a monthly subscription fee to keep health insurance. (Example: if your policy has a $300 monthly premium, you need to pay the company $300 per month to stay covered.)
- **Claim**: what a medical professional tells your insurance company they did for you. Claims can be paid or "denied", meaning the insurance company wants to not pay for those goods and services.
- **Covered** or **coverage**: maintaining the possibility that your insurance company will pay for some of your medical care's costs. Also what-

ever goods and services your insurance company will pay for. And what they give you permission to use and who they give you permission to see. (Example: if your policy says a colonscopy with Dr. Y is covered, they will pay some or all of the price Dr. Y charges them. But remember: you still have to "meet" your yearly deductible before they pay for anything.)

• **Provider**: a medical professional or facility who can help. (Example: Your policy might list Dr. Z as a covered provider and ABC Hospital as a covered provider.)

• **Explanation of Benefits**: a document meant to show you claims your insurance paid for and claims they didn't. These documents are notoriously hard to understand (by design!), so you can call your insurance company and ask for explanations and/or a "detailed Explanation of Benefits."

• **Formulary**: the list of drugs the company will or won't pay for. (Example: your policy's formulary lists each drug they'll pay for and puts them in categories or classes. Those categories/classes refer to what portion of a drug's price they'll cover.)

• **Maximum out-of-pocket**: the maximum amount of money the company will expect you to pay for covered medical goods and services each year (insert a hundred asterisks here). Sometimes companies won't count coinsurance charges in this number, they'll never count premiums in this number, and there might be other loopholes and surprises, so try to get clear definitions of your maximum out-of-pocket from representatives of your health insurance company. (Example: if your policy has a maximum out-of-pocket of $15,000, they'll pay any medical charge over $15,000 for covered goods and services. But remember: this figure can be misleading.)

- **HMO**: Health Maintenance Organization. A health insurance plan that usually covers fewer providers than PPO's and requires you to work with a primary care physician. Often cheaper than PPO plans.
- **PPO**: Preferred Provider Organization. A health insurance plan that usually covers more providers and services than HMO's. Often more expensive than HMO's.
- **Out-of-network**: a medical facility or professional your insurance company doesn't want to pay for. (Example: Your policy's website doesn't list Dr. B as a covered physician. Dr. B is out-of-network.)

RULE OF THUMB #9: Make people define their terms. Medical and insurance professionals talk in jargon. Ask them to repeat themselves and define words that are confusing.

FINDING A PLAN

If you don't have coverage through your job and don't qualify for Medicare or Medicaid, you'll need to find a plan through your state's Affordable Care Act marketplace. (Medicare is a health insurance plan run by the federal government which primarily covers folks 65 years old or older. Medicaid is a health insurance program run by federal and state governments, and it covers mostly low-income folks and people with disabilities.)

Translation: go to healthcare.gov and follow instructions there to buy coverage. That site will tell you if you qualify for your state's Medicaid plan.

Health insurance companies are legally required to offer plans in these state marketplaces, but you can only buy coverage during a "qualifying life event." [healthcare.gov/glossary/qualifying-life-event] There are four types of these events:

1. Loss of health coverage
2. Changes in household
3. Changes in residence
4. Other qualifying events (often changes in income or citizenship status)

When you're looking at plans, make sure they cover your medications and the nearest hospital in which you'd like to be treated. Also, make sure the plans cover doctors you'd like to work with. You can do this with healthcare.gov's search filters.

Next, evaluate plans with your finances in

mind. I usually focus on maximum out-of-pocket numbers, speciality drug coverage, deductible amounts, and co-insurance amounts. Remember that the federal government might pay some or all of your monthly premiums depending on your income, so provide accurate info about your income to healthcare.gov.

RULE OF THUMB #10: Don't buy bad insurance. It's better to pay known amounts now than unknown amounts later. Medical bills are the USA's most common cause of bankruptcy. Sign up for the best plan you can afford.

USING YOUR COVERAGE

Once you have coverage, put printed copies of your health insurance membership cards in your wallet. I also recommend keeping digital copies on your phone and computer.

The back of these cards usually have a phone number you can call to ask questions and get info.

Receptionists in medical offices will scan your insurance cards before your appointments and tell you if you owe a co-pay.

Pharmacists will do the same thing. Sometimes it'll be cheaper to buy a drug without "applying" your insurance coverage, so ask your pharmacists if this is the case for your purchase.

Now let's imagine two different scenarios:

Let's call the first scenario **No Bullshit**. It's January 5th. You've just visited the ER and spent three nights in a shared hospital room. You knew before going that your plan covers this hospital. You go home with a diagnosis, some prescriptions, and a followup appointment.

Two weeks later you get your first piece of mail from the hospital. It says "$35,468" on it.

You don't panic because you remember not all documents from hospitals are bills and that all medical bills are negotiable.

The piece of paper shows that your insurance paid the hospital $30,468 for various goods and services. The "amount owed"—what you're expected to pay the hospital—is $5,000.

If your deductible for covered ("in-network") major medical services is $5,000, then this number makes sense.

You call the hospital, negotiate the bill down, and set up a payment plan.

It's expensive, but you've read this book so there are no surprises.

Let's call the second scenario **Bullshit**.

Same setup: an ER visit followed by three nights in the in-network hospital.

You're healing up at home when you get a bill in the mail. It says that you owe them $30,468. Your insurance only paid the hospital $5,000.

A week after that, you get an Explanation of Benefits document from your insurance. It's confusing. A little asterisk points to tiny print that says "AN OUT-OF-NETWORK PROVIDER OR FACILITY PROVIDED THESE SERVICES." Part of your claim has been denied.

And the EOB is a mess. You can't make sense of what the hospital charged your insurance; you can't tell what exactly the insurance company paid for and what they didn't. Some numbers are duplicated; some charges seem to conflict with others. The dates are wrong.

And yet you're supposed to pay the hospital over $30,000.

Now what?

FIGHTING THE BULLSHIT

Documents from insurance companies more often contain bullshit than clarity.

Here's how I recommend reacting to health insurance companies' bullshit: first, if you're angry, do something with that anger. Scream, punch something soft, exercise, lift something heavy and throw it across the room. Whatever. Just convert that anger into action.

Then sit down with the bullshit document and take notes on it. What's confusing? What seems incorrect? Write out your thoughts and make annotations.

Then convert your notes into simple statements and questions you can use during your phonecalls with your health insurance company.

Here are some examples, using the Bullshit situation above:

- "Your company was billed for a procedure that took place on January 1st, but I wasn't in the hospital until January 3rd. Please explain this."
- "It looks like your company paid part of this claim, but then I was billed twice for the same procedure. Why?"
- "This EOB says that your company paid for the antibiotics I was prescribed, but not the saline solution used for that IV. How does that make any sense?"

After writing down those sentences and questions, take a day or two to just go about your life, relax, and try to get a clear head. Schedule 1–2 hours during the week to sit down and call your insurance company or the providers. Make sure you make these calls on a full stomach.

During these calls, be as nice as possible, but use anger as a tool. Write everything down. Try to talk with people with fancier-sounding job titles. Make the representatives on the phone define their terms and explain things clearly. Finally, value your time: if handling an issue is taking a long time and you'd rather just pay the bill and be done with it, do that.

If the last paragraph looks familiar, that's because it contains most of the Rules of Thumb I've outlined so far. Why? Because having phone conversations with insurance company representatives and providers is sadly a big part of being sick in the United States of America. You can and should bring all your skills and knowledge to these conversations. Sometimes your medicine, your treatment, or your financial stability will depend on it.

Finally, if your health insurance company denies a claim, you can appeal their decision.

Appealing a denied claim or cancelled coverage can seem overwhelming, but it isn't complicated. You'll need to fill out forms, send letters and/or emails, and make some calls. (For more details about the process, check out healthcare.gov/appeal-insurance-company-decision/appeals)

You'll need to make the best argument you can because you're trying to convince your insurance company that they should spend money they don't want to spend. The more evidence you can use, and the more precise that evidence is, the better. If you can get a statement from your doctor supporting your appeal, do it. If you find any contradictions or misleading statements in your insurance policy, quote them.

When appealing a health insurance company's bullshit, it might help to imagine you're the lead in a TV series about the world's best lawyer. (I'm not joking!) Or, for basketball fans, imagine you're Michael Jordan and the insurance company is that rookie who talked shit about your ability on the court.

Like Mike or that all-star lawyer, dominate

them in and on the court.

If your insurance company still denies your claim or denies your coverage, don't give up. You can still request an "external review", meaning the insurance company's decision and all the info behind it is sent to a third party for a final determination.

RULE OF THUMB #11: Fight paperwork with paperwork. Insurance companies try to confuse you with their paperwork because they profit off your confusion. Hit them with clear arguments, direct quotes, and tons of evidence.

COVERING YOUR ASS

We live in a country in which some married couples get divorced so that the sick partner can be covered by Medicaid instead of unaffordable private insurance plans. This is a sad truth about the USA.

Any nation worth a damn should make sure all its residents can fearlessly get the care and medicine they need to heal and stay healthy. We're not one of those nations.

Because of this, I recommend that everyone make sure they have health insurance. Surviving a medical emergency is stressful enough; no one needs to deal with hundreds of thousands of dollars of bills, calls from debt collectors, and ruined credit scores because an illness or accident happened to them. If you have health insurance—public or private—you're protecting yourself, at least partially, from terrible financial consequences.

To qualify for and keep Medicaid coverage, you'll need to limit your yearly income. How much you can make depends on your state. Usually you'll need to make no more than 138% of the federal poverty level each year to keep Medicaid coverage.

In 2021, for one person, this is $17,774.40 (which is 138% of $12,880). For two people, it's $24,039.60 (138% of $17,420). All these amounts can be found here: kff.org/health-reform/state-indicator/medicaid-income-eligibility-limits-for-adults-as-a-percent-of-the-federal-poverty-level

If you don't qualify for Medicaid, you can stay covered by a private insurance plan offered through healthcare.gov. The federal government will pay a percentage of your monthly premiums based on your income; the less you make, the more they pay. Even with this help, though, some won't be able to afford these plans.

The other option for sick people in the United States is to work: by working, they can keep employer-sponsored health insurance (a.k.a. "group plans"). Many chronically ill people here must choose to live in poverty or work as if they were healthy. The other option is to marry someone whose employer offers health insurance, becoming your new spouse's dependent.

Employers who offer group plans either deduct their plan's monthly premiums from your paychecks, pay some of those premiums, or pay all of them. If you're covered by a group plan, talk with workers in your job's Human Resources department to learn more about your coverage.

If you're fired or if your hours are reduced, you might have to use COBRA. COBRA is a law that allows folks who've lost their coverage in these circumstances to stay covered for between 18 and 36 months. This coverage is usually more expensive, but sometimes it's wise to keep it while you look for coverage elsewhere. You can learn more about COBRA here: dol.gov/sites/dolgov/files/EBSA/about-ebsa/our-activities/resource-center/faqs/cobra-continuation-health-coverage-consumer.pdf

LIFE

A baby needs milk, warmth, and touch. Adults need sleep, food, water, and relationships. Trees need sunshine; bees need flowers. Need is fundamental to life.

As a sick person, you're going to experience frustration and sadness. You'll feel disappointed with your body. You'll regret your choices. You'll feel exhausted with how exhausted you are. You probably will resent the fact that you need medicine and care in order to survive.

But you must to do your best to love yourself for your needs, not in spite of them.

Our political and economic system brainwashes us into thinking that people who need help are burdensome. As a sick person, you need to overcome this brainwashing. As a sick person you must learn to love yourself, to accept yourself, no matter how useless you feel. This is a survival skill.

RULE OF THUMB #12: Try loving yourself. Our culture is cruel to the weak, poor, and sick. One way you can heal up from the stress of that cruelty is to practice accepting your needs and loving yourself for them.

LIMITS

Getting sick when you've been mostly healthy is a shocking experience. Your life changes profoundly because the range of actions available to you every day dramatically shrinks. Getting sick limits your world.

And in order to heal up from most illnesses, you need to learn the terrain of this smaller world. What does that mean practically? You need to learn how to do less. Much less. You need to learn how to rest, how to say no, and how to limit your activity.

This can be very frustrating, particularly for busy people. But limiting your commitments and responsibilities while you're sick is incredibly important. Not only will you need to rest more in order to heal, but being chronically ill can make your life unpredictable in new ways. Before getting sick, maybe you could safely promise to meet up with friends every Friday night after work. After getting sick, you might have to keep your nights free so that you can respect what your body's telling you.

And believe me: your body (including your mind) will let you know what it can and cannot do—with pain, with fatigue, with nausea, with anxiety, etc. Respecting that information is the hard part.

Learn to say no. A trick I recommend is responding to invitations with this phrase: "That sounds fun but I need to play it by ear. Will you follow up with me the day of?" This lets you not make a promise you might not be able to keep while keeping open the option of attending, if your health permits it.

If you're chronically ill, you might have to rethink your career and ambitions. This can be a deeply painful process. Part of being a sick person is accepting that you have dignity and worth even if you can't work fulltime, or make art, or support your family financially, or pursue your hobbies. You've got to make peace with just existing—because when you're really sick, that might be all you're able to do until you heal up.

FEAR

This is a scary country. It's a violent country. It's a great place if you're rich, but it can be brutally difficult if you're not.

Fear is a powerful emotion, and it's one that sick people feel all the time in the United States of America. We're afraid of medical emergencies. We're afraid of having to stay in the hospital. We're afraid of medical bills. We're afraid of not being able to afford our prescriptions. We're afraid of losing our jobs, our health insurance. Fear seems like it's everywhere.

I want you to know that it's okay to be afraid. Why? Because fear tells us that something can be better.

We could easily improve our country's health care systems. We could improve and expand public health insurance programs. We could limit drug prices. We could pass laws that help workers who've been laid off. We could provide paid sick leave to everyone. All these possibilities are real—they just require political will, time, and good organizing.

Fear, then, is related to hope.

HOPE

I want you to practice asking for help.

Hopefully you've already started practicing. If you've asked a friend or family member to read this book or stay with you in the hospital, that's a great start.

Keep practicing. Ask for help understanding your diagnosis. Ask for help getting to your next doctor's appointment. Ask for help with the groceries. Ask for help remembering to take your medicine. Ask for financial help. Practice this skill, because the reality is this: when we're sick, we need help to live. And that's okay.

I want you to ask for help because asking for help is the most beautiful thing in the world.

Thank you. I pray that you're healing.

RULES OF THUMB

1: Ask someone you trust to help. Having someone who can advocate for you, listen, and guide your decisions will make your life as a sick person much easier.

2: Write everything down. Whenever you talk with someone who has power over your health and finances, write down their name, contact info, the date, and what they say. You can use this info later to protect yourself.

3: Be nice, but use anger as a tool. Sadly, anger can more effectively get you attention from people with power. As a sick person, though, anger can make you sicker—so use it wisely.

4: Work with people with fancier-sounding job titles. They have more power and information so they can help you more efficiently. Keep their contact info handy.

5: Bills are negotiable. They're made by people

and people can be persuaded to change their minds. Don't panic.

6: Don't pay medical bills immediately. Bills say how long you have to pay them (it's usually 30, 60, or 90 days). First understand and negotiate those charges and prices.

7: Value your time. Waiting on hold for hours can be as harmful as a disease's symptoms, so figure out what your time is worth per hour. Use that number to choose which bills you fight.

8: When in doubt, take your time. If your condition allows you to, research drugs and their risks, ask questions, and make a careful and deliberate decision.

9: Make people define their terms. Medical and insurance professionals talk in jargon. Ask them to repeat themselves and define words that are confusing.

10: Don't buy bad insurance. It's better to pay known amounts now than unknown amounts later. Medical bills are the USA's most common cause of bankruptcy. Sign up for the best plan you can afford.

11: Fight paperwork with paperwork. Insurance companies try to confuse you with their paperwork because they profit off your confusion. Hit them with clear arguments, direct quotes, and tons of evidence.

12: Try loving yourself. Our culture is cruel to the weak, poor, and sick. One way you can heal up from the stress of that cruelty is to practice accepting your needs and loving yourself for them.

RESOURCES

Finding health insurance
healthcare.gov

Paying for treatment
copays.org
panfoundation.org
benefits.gov

Finding a doctor
doctor.webmd.com

Finding support groups
mayoclinic.org/healthy-lifestyle/stress-management/in-depth/support-groups/art-20044655
nami.org/Support-Education/Support-Groups

If you're struggling with suicidal thoughts
1-800-273-8255
suicidepreventionlifeline.org/chat

www.ingramcontent.com/pod-product-compliance
Lightning Source LLC
Chambersburg PA
CBHW070038070426
42449CB00012BA/3085